THE COLORFUL SMOOTHIES BOOK

Clarice Cameron

Copyright © 2022 by Clarice Cameron

All rights reserved.

No portion of this book may be reproduced in any form without written permission from the publisher or author, except as permitted by U.S. copyright law.

Contents

1. Introduction   1

2. Smoothies Are Good For You For
    These 10 Reasons   6

3. Convenient Substitutes and Nutritious
    Ingredients   24

4. Diabetes and Loss of Pounds   54

5. Dietary Supplementation   82

6. Lovely recipes   100

7. Super easy   134

8. The lasts   147

Chapter One

Introduction

It is not uncommon to hear about "miracle" dietary promises that fall short of the mark when tested in the real world. Then there's the ever-present smoothie. If you're looking for a way to boost your health by eating more fruits and vegetables, you might want to look elsewhere. The addition of smoothies to my daily diet boosted my athleticism and health to new heights.

It was in graduate school in Fort Collins, Colorado, where I was studying for a master's de-

2   THE COLORFUL SMOOTHIES BOOK

gree in nutrition and exercise science and to become a registered dietitian, that I first discovered my passion for smoothies. I was also training hard with one of the top coaches in the country and competed in several 10Ks, half marathons, marathons, and triathlons, as well as prepping for a half marathon. As a novice vegetarian, I was still learning the ins and outs of a well-rounded diet. I must admit, there were a few areas in which I might have done better; for example, my post-training recuperation and energy levels could have been better. A new smoothie bar at Alfalfa's Market caught my eye when I was working there part-time. I'd never had a smoothie before, but my coworkers persuaded me to try it. Strawberry Fields, Blue Diva, and CaColorado, to mention a few, were my favourites. And what's more, there's more! They were just amazing! Sweet and nutrient-dense, this pudding is thick and creamy.

INTRODUCTION 3

I was astonished at how much better I felt after taking them. "Supercharged" is how I felt. Recovering from lengthy runs and speed work was much improved on the days I drank smoothies. Making smoothies got me hooked on eating them, so I started experimenting on my own at home with a variety of fruits and other components.

Smoothie making is a great way to boost your nutrition because they can be made with a wide variety of ingredients. Probiotics, omega-3s, grains, legumes, nuts, and phytochemical-rich foods may all be added to smoothies to boost their nutritional value. They may be used as a nutritious breakfast, a post-workout recovery drink, a light lunch, or a filling afternoon snack, to name just a few of its many uses.

4   THE COLORFUL SMOOTHIES BOOK

I've been playing around with smoothie "bowls" recently. Instead of sipping smoothies with a straw, you may use them to eat them with a spoon. Toppings such as granola, hemp seeds, or slices of nuts are common in smoothie bowls, which are thicker in substance. If you're like me and prefer eating out of bowls, smoothie bowls could be a fun alternative to conventional smoothies.

If you try the recipes in this book, I hope you'll become a regular smoothie drinker.

Smoothies Made to Order for Optimum Well-Being

Eating healthily on a budget and with enough time to spare can be difficult. Increasingly, Americans are eating on the move, snatching a bite to eat between work, children's activities, and other activities that keep them busy from dawn to

INTRODUCTION   5

night.. When it comes to convenience foods, artificial chemicals, fat, sugar, and salt are commonly found in commercially produced items meant for on-the-go consumption. These low-cost, quick-to-prepare foods are low in nutritional value. Without the vitamins and minerals needed to maintain excellent health, these meals may be a decent source of calories but nothing more. • Let's get a smoothie going! The smoothies in this book are rich with vitamins and minerals, yet they don't bust your caloric or cost budgets. They're quick and cheap to cook, and they're a great supper or snack to have on hand while you're on the go.

Chapter Two

Smoothies Are Good For You For These 10 Reasons

Smoothies are a great way to improve your health. The health benefits of smoothies, if you've never tried them, are about to be revealed to you.

The first step is to eat more fruits and vegetables each day. A study published in the Journal of the Academy of Nutrition and Dietetics found that the majority of Americans did not meet the daily recommendations for fruit and vegetable con-

SMOOTHIES ARE GOOD FOR YOU FOR..7

sumption at all. Smoothies are an excellent way to get your daily servings of fruits and vegetables.

There is more diversity in your diet. When it comes to consuming nutritious food that you don't particularly like, smoothies are an excellent vehicle for doing so. In the case of superfood kale, mixing it with fruits in a smoothie can mask its taste while still providing the nutritional advantages of this dark, leafy green, such as iron, calcium, and magnesium.

You increase the amount of fibre in your diet. The Mayo Clinic recommends that women have around 25 grammes of fibre per day, while men should consume about 35 grammes per day. Around 15 grammes is all that Americans eat on a daily basis. Fiber is critical to overall health since it aids digestion, fills you up, and protects your heart. You can get closer to the guidelines by

8   THE COLORFUL SMOOTHIES BOOK

using fibre fruits, vegetables, and seeds (like flax or chia) in your smoothies.

You up your consumption of antioxidants. Antioxidants can help minimise cell damage that comes about from oxidative stress. Antioxidant-rich foods like fruits and vegetables may help lower the chance of getting certain illnesses when consumed.

You eat more fruits and vegetables. Your vitamin and mineral intake will be substantially improved even by substituting one or two fast or processed food meals each week with smoothies. Fruits and vegetables in smoothies are nutrient-dense, but those in processed and fast-food meals are not.

You cut back on the amount of additional sugars you eat. Added sugar is a major source of extra calories and no nutritional value in the American diet. Having a sugar-free smoothie instead of a

SMOOTHIES ARE GOOD FOR YOU FOR..9

sweet snack is a terrific way to cut down on the amount of sugar you consume in your diet.

7. Salt intake is decreased. About 75% of salt intake comes from processed and fast meals, according to the American Heart Association; swapping these for healthier, less salted alternatives like smoothies may help lower the risk of high blood pressure.

You're less stressed out in general. When making smoothies a regular part of your diet, you'll be less likely to suffer the effects of stress. It's not the ingredients in smoothies that are responsible for this, but rather the lifestyle changes that smoothies will have on your body. Smoothies can help you save money and time since they are so quick and simple to make. Making and drinking smoothies might become a part of your regular routine.

10   THE COLORFUL SMOOTHIES BOOK

You eat less food. Using smoothies instead of fast food or processed food can help you lose weight, depending on the smoothies you select. Choosing low-fat, low-calorie components and healthy fruits and vegetables might help you replace a few high-calorie meals a week with smoothies.

You increase the range of nutrients you include in your diet. Vitamins and minerals may be found in the food you consume, but it's not always possible to create nutritious meals every day. Smoothies come in handy in this situation. When you're on the go and don't have time to make a typical meal, smoothies are a great option because they can be easily supplemented with nutrition-enhancing powders and liquids.

The beautiful thing about this book's smoothie recipes is that they're so easy to tweak and change to suit your needs. Substitute ideas are

SMOOTHIES ARE GOOD FOR YOU FOR.11

included in the recipes, but you may also experiment on your own. Building your own smoothies with the help of this book's charts and tables will allow you to create mixtures that are tailored to your specific nutritional needs.

A non-dairy alternative to milk can be used to make a dairy-free smoothie, for example. If you're concerned about calories, choose for items that are lower in calories or fat content, such as vegetables. Spice up your smoothie by adding one of the spices listed in the list below. What ever you decide, this book makes it simple to alter any smoothie's taste or texture or nutritional or fat content in any way you like. Take the recipe as a starting point and modify it to meet your own requirements.

The Basics of Making a Smoothie

12 THE COLORFUL SMOOTHIES BOOK

You would think that making a smoothie is as simple as throwing everything in a blender and blending until smooth. This method may work on occasion, but if you want a delicious and nutritious smoothie every time, follow this simple 7-step process.

Select a dish from the menu. Make a strategy before you start cooking, so choose a dish based on your health objectives and follow the recipe labelled in this book. Prepare and assemble your ingredients ahead of time.

Add the liquid you want to use. Use the blender's blades as a guide and add liquid until the tips are covered with roughly a cup of liquid. Add more liquid if you like your smoothies to be thinner, and less if you prefer them to be thicker.

Add to your foundation. The "body" or "base" of your smoothie will give it a creamy consistency,

SMOOTHIES ARE GOOD FOR YOU FOR.13

mass, and a flavour of its own. Adding a base to your smoothie is a great way to increase its nutritional value and provide a source of protein. Bananas, mangos, and peaches, which are creamy and sweet, are excellent basis. Other healthy possibilities are avocados, nut butters, tofu, yoghurt, chia seed gel, cooked beans, and oats.

Add fruits and/or veggies. Besides sweetness and texture, fruits also provide nutrients including fibre and vitamins. You may use fresh or frozen fruit in most recipes, so play around and find what works best for you. Add greens like spinach or kale to your diet and experiment with fruit and vegetable pairings to see what works best for you.

Optional add-ons. You may add nutrients and taste to your smoothie in this part of the process. spices, protein powders and superfoods such as blueberries and spinach can be added to the mix.

14 THE COLORFUL SMOOTHIES BOOK

Blend until the mixture is completely smooth. When you're ready to go faster, go for it on the slowest setting first (if you have one). Blend for about 10 seconds, or until the liquid is completely circulating. Blending duration might range from 30 to 60 seconds, depending on the type of components and your personal choice.

Take a sip. As a last step, be sure to use a big container and serve immediately.

Adding a Little Spice

Adding a little kick to your smoothie is a great idea. You are not the only one. In recent years, the use of spices in smoothies has grown in popularity. Spices are prized by some for the flavour they contribute to smoothies, while others look for specific health advantages in order to enhance their smoothies' nutritional value. Here are some ideas to get you started.

SMOOTHIES ARE GOOD FOR YOU FOR.15

ALLSPICE

Aroma: warm, somewhat sweet, a little pungent, and spicy.

TREATMENT FOR GAS AND INFLUENZA:

Suggested serving size: 1/8 teaspoon PAIRINGS: fruit, pumpkin, and winter squash

ANISE

TASTE: A sweet licorice note

HEALTH BENEFITS: Expectorant, diuretic, and gas-relieving properties.

Suggested serving size: 1/8 teaspoon FRUIT AND APPLES

CARDAMOM

TASTE: Spicy, sweet, and sour

THE COLORFUL SMOOTHIES BOOK

DIGESTIVE ASSISTANCE, HEARTBURN TREATMENT, and GAS TREATMENT:

Aphrodisiac, analgesic, and thermogenic properties are among the health benefits of cayenne.

TOTAL RECOMMENDED QUANTITY: a couple of grains

A wide variety of foods can be paired with each other: fruits and vegetables, nuts and seeds.

CINNAMBI (not cassia cinnamon)

TASTE: Spicy, mildly sweet, and warm

Nutritional benefits include antioxidants, anti-inflammatory properties, the potential to enhance lipid profiles, as well as an increased ability to regulate blood sugar levels.

14 teaspoon is a good starting point.

SMOOTHIES ARE GOOD FOR YOU FOR.17

Most fruits, berries, nuts, and seeds may be paired together.

CLOVES

TASTE: sweet, bitter, and sour

HEALTH VALUE: expectorant, calming stomach discomfort, toothache

Suggested serving size: 1/8 teaspoon

Apples, beets, pears, pumpkin, root vegetables, and squash are some of the best pairings.

CORIANDER

TASTING NOTES: A citrusy, somewhat bitter flavour.

Nutritional value: gastrointestinal tonic, flatulence, irritable bowel syndrome.

14 teaspoon is a good starting point. Combinations: Banana-Apple-Citrus

18 THE COLORFUL SMOOTHIES BOOK

CUMIN

TASTE: Spicy, heated, pungent, with a harsh aftertaste

Digestive tonic, diuretic, and diarrheal

A quarter of a teaspoon

fruits and vegetables including avocados, oranges, coconuts, and cucumbers

FENNEL

TASTE: licorice-like sweetness

Treats indigestion and gas, and relieves a cough.

Suggested serving size: 1/8 to 1/4 teaspoon

COMPANIONS: apple, celery, pears, bananas and berries.

FENUGREEK

SMOOTHIES ARE GOOD FOR YOU FOR.19

Warm, somewhat sweet, and mildly nutty, with a hint of maple

An anti-inflammatory and digestive help, as well as an improvement in blood lipids.

Suggested serving size: 1/8 teaspoon

PAIRINGS: apple, pears, bananas, squash, and pumpkin

GINGER

TASTE: peppery, sweet, woody, and hot

Treats nausea, digestive tonic, fights heartburn, expectorant value

14 teaspoon is a good starting point.

PAIRINGS: squash, root vegetables, apples, pears, citrus, banana, cucumber

MACE

THE COLORFUL SMOOTHIES BOOK

FLAVOR: similar to nutmeg, but less potent

It has antibacterial and anti-inflammatory properties.

14 teaspoon is a good starting point.

PAIRINGS: berries, pumpkin, and spinach

NUTMEG

TASTE: peppery, sweet, and smoky.

PREMIUM VALUE: anti-inflammatory, antibacterial, and antioxidant

A quarter of a teaspoon

a wide variety of vegetables and fruits

PEPPERCORN

(black, white, pink, and green) are some of the colours that are available.

TASTE: peppery, smoky, and warming

SMOOTHIES ARE GOOD FOR YOU FOR.21

ENVIRONMENTAL BENEFITS: expectorant, thermogenic

Suggested serving size: 1/8 to 1/4 teaspoon Vegetables and fruits go well together.

TURMERIC

Bitter and spicy like mild ginger but much more intense.

Anti-inflammatory and antioxidant properties

Suggested serving size: 1/8 teaspoon TREAT COMBINATIONS: citrus and root veggies

Coffee with a hint of vanilla

Sweet and moderate in flavour

Treats bloating and gas.

1/4 to 1/2 teaspoon is a good starting point. Suggested food pairings: a wide variety of fruits, nuts, and seeds.

22   THE COLORFUL SMOOTHIES BOOK

The Charts of Contrasts

With the aid of the Mix-and-Match charts in this part, you may come up with an endless number of smoothie concoctions. You may play around with different fruits and veggies to see what works for you.

Your personal tastes and the ratios of frozen, fresh, and liquid components will determine whether or not you utilise ice. For a thinner shake, use 1 to 4 cubes, while for a thicker drink, use 5 to 10 cubes. There are no hard and fast rules when it comes to making a 16-ounce smoothie, so experiment to find what works best for you.

Flavors and textures may be mixed and matched in any way you choose.

Do you want your smoothies sweet and slushie-style? Is this dessert sweet and spongy?

SMOOTHIES ARE GOOD FOR YOU FOR 23

Perhaps you like a little less sweetness and a little more spiciness in your food. Use the chart in this section to identify what you like. '

Chapter Three

Convenient Substitutes and Nutritious Ingredients

As you practise preparing smoothies, you'll get more familiar with the various components and be able to make quick and easy replacements. To assist you pick substitute ingredients if you don't have what a recipe calls for on hand, the following Mix-and-Match chart is provided. Smoothies may be made with just about any beverage, but sugary fruit juices should be avoided. Instead, choose for 100% juice or make your own. Adding creaminess may be achieved by using milk, but

CONVENIENT SUBSTITUTES AND NUTRI...

filtered water is a healthier alternative if you don't mind the liquid's taste interfering with your drink.

Banana, mango, peach, pears, apples, and papaya are all examples of "creamy" fruits to include in your diet. Banana and strawberry, apple and blueberry, and mango and pineapple are all excellent pairings. Greens like spinach, which have little to no flavour, can be added to smoothies to improve nutrients and thicken them. To prevent producing a "sugar explosion," include at least one protein and one healthy fat.

Experiment with different ingredients to give your dish a unique look, feel, and flavour.

Troubleshooting Smoothie Problems

There are times when your smoothie doesn't turn out the way you expected it to, regardless of how experienced you are at making them. Do you

THE COLORFUL SMOOTHIES BOOK

throw it in the trash, waste the ingredients, get irritated, and write it off as a "live and learn" lesson, or do you save it and try again? If that's the case, are you up to the task of making the best smoothie you've ever had? For me, food waste is a no-no, therefore I choose to take up the task and encourage others to do the same.

COLOR THAT DOESN'T GO WELL WITH OTHERS

Because we eat with our eyes as much as our mouths, a brown smoothie may wind up in the compost pile despite the fact that it has no effect on the vitamin and mineral content. Spinach, kale, broccoli, cucumber, and mint can be paired with green, yellow, or orange fruits like kiwifruit, pears, green apples, pineapples, mangos, and apricots to keep your smoothie green.

CONVENIENT SUBSTITUTES AND NUTRI... CREATED WITH A WATERY OR LIGHT CONSISTENCY

A number of smoothie components rate among the most magical in the world of nutrition. Xanthan gum and guar gum will solve all of your watery smoothie woes. Gums may thicken your smoothie without adding extra calories, carbs, or lipids because they are vegan and gluten-free. Gums are excellent thickening agents, and a small amount goes a long way. Smoothies can benefit from the addition of either xanthan or guar gum, but combining the two yields the best results because of their apparent synergy. To begin, use 12 teaspoon of each, or 1 teaspoon if you're just utilising one. Add the gums to the blender with the rest of the ingredients and blend until smooth. Frozen bananas, oats, nut butters, tofu, milk, and yoghurt are all excellent thickeners if you don't mind the extra calories. Chia seeds, which create a gel when soaked in water for a few minutes, are another fantastic alternative. Add them to your liquid, let them sit for approximately 15 minutes, and then add the rest of the ingredients to the mixture.

The CONSISTENCY IS EITHER GROUND OR CHUNKY

You may need to mix it for a few more seconds to smooth out any chunks. Large chunks of fruit and veggies may break apart if your blender isn't powerful enough to handle complete components like dates. Precutting or grinding big items in a food processor before adding to your smoothie is the best answer in this scenario. If your smoothie has a gritty texture, it's possible that you used too much protein powder. You may want to experiment with half of the suggested serving size until

CONVENIENT SUBSTITUTES AND NUT... 29

you discover a protein powder with a flavour and texture you like.

THICKNESS OF INTEGRITY

Add additional milk to your smoothie to thin it out without diluting the flavour (cow, plant-, or nut-based). To get the correct consistency, add 12 cup at a time at first. Avoid using water to thin out a smoothie since it will dilute the flavour and you'll have two issues to deal with at once.

BITTERNESS

Solution: Arugula and dandelion greens, both of which have a bitter flavour, can overshadow a smoothie. Instead of using a bitter fruit or vegetable, try using a sweet fruit or vegetable to mask the bitterness first. Bananas, spinach, and fruit like strawberries, pineapples, and mangoes can help to mask unpleasant flavours. A couple of

30 THE COLORFUL SMOOTHIES BOOK

these substances can be kept frozen and used to neutralise off-putting tastes.

SWEETNESS

A simple solution to a sugar-laden smoothie is to double-check your components. Sweeteners may convert your plant- and nut-based milk into a sugar bomb, as can most yoghurts and protein powders. In order to lessen the sweetness of the mixture, you can include a taste neutralizer such as half a banana, some avocado, some frozen spinach, some lemon juice, or even a few slices of pear. If it doesn't work, a pinch of salt will do the trick.

BAD TASTE OR SWEETNESS

Fortunately, most smoothie recipes contain enough fruit to sweeten them without the need for added sugar. Some smoothie enthusiasts

CONVENIENT SUBSTITUTES AND NUTRI...

favour Medjool dates as the greatest way to sweeten a smoothie organically when that isn't the case, however The caramel-like flavour of these dates makes them a great addition to any smoothie. Unless you have a high-powered blender, you may simply chop up the fruit and throw it in with the others. In the absence of soaking dates in warm water and chopping them into little pieces, you can just add them to your liquid foundation. Overripe bananas plus a tiny amount of stevia, honey, or maple syrup can also be used as natural sweeteners.

substituting fresh or frozen food

Because fresh fruits and veggies don't have the same consistency as frozen ones, you'll need to use thicker ones to make your smoothie thicker. Instead of using water, go for a dairy product like yoghurt or tofu; sprinkle in seeds like chia and

32 THE COLORFUL SMOOTHIES BOOK

xanthan gum; and add a few additional cubes to the mix. Replace ice with water and modify the quantities of the heavier items you use if you only have frozen fruits and veggies on hand.

Using the Recipes and Understanding the Labels

The recipes in this book are divided up into sections depending on their nutritional value, which is reflected in the chapter headings. Recipes for weight loss, cleansing, and anti-inflammatory smoothies are just a few of the topics covered. In the same way, the labels on the recipes help you figure out how they'll work with different diets. You may use the index at the back of the book to search for recipes by name or ingredient. There are a number of ways to categorise the recipes.

Cleanse and detoxify your body.

CONVENIENT SUBSTITUTES AND NUTR...

Toxins and environmental pollutants are removed and cleansed from the body through the process of "detoxification," which is short for "detoxification." Excessively low-calorie detox diets might leave you feeling weak and exhausted for days or even weeks. They might potentially be harmful.. Regular exercise, plenty of water, and daily detoxification smoothies are a better way to get your body in shape and keep it healthy. Lemons, cilantro, watermelon, ginger, dandelion greens, green tea, kale, avocado, apples, beets, yoghurt, and more are all included in this chapter's dishes. Cleansing components are plentiful when it comes to incorporating them into smoothies. Most have a pleasant flavour, while others can be easily disguised by more strongly flavoured components. Try out these dishes and incorporate them into your daily diet. Detox di-

34   THE COLORFUL SMOOTHIES BOOK

ets that severely restrict your caloric intake are avoided this way.

Spinach Cleanser with Lemon and Lime

Lemon and lime are two of the most common detox ingredients, and they work together to create a pleasant and purifying smoothie. citrus fruits are abundant in vitamin C, which can promote digestion, stimulate the liver and aid in the evacuation of waste. Potassium-rich bananas receive a fibre and chlorophyll boost from spinach in this alkalizing dish.

1 cup of water.

1-half a lemon, seeded and de-pitted

A seeded and peeled half lime

1 medium sliced frozen banana

Spinach florets in 2 cups

CONVENIENT SUBSTITUTES AND NUTRI...

To 1 cup ice, add 1 pitted Medjool date12

There are optional add-ons:

12-cup bagged blueberries in the freezer

12 tbsp. freshly grated ginger

Amount of avocado: 2 Tablespoons

Blend all of the ingredients together until they're completely dissolved. Serve as soon as possible.

For a smoothie that is thicker and more flavorful, use frozen spinach rather than raw spinach. Frozen veggies are a fantastic alternative for decreasing food waste since they are prepared at their highest nutritional value.

Counts as one serving; serving size is one Calories: 177; Total Fat: 1; SUGAR: 24; SODIUM: 50; CARBOHYDRATES: 46; FIBER 7; PROTEIN: 4;

Endive Peachy in Flavor

The same old spinach or kale smoothies have you bored to tears? Instead, try endive! Endive is a natural diuretic that can help you maintain a healthy digestive tract and improve intestinal regularity. The earthy bitterness of the endive pairs beautifully with the fruity sweetness of the peach and mango in this nourishing and energising smoothie.

1 litre of coconut water

12 cup of mango that has been frozen

0.5 lbs. peaches frozen Endive juice made with 2 cups of endive and 14 of a lemon

1 tsp. flaxseed meal

12 to 1 cup ice, 1 tablespoon chia seeds

There are optional add-ons:

12 ice-cold bananas

CONVENIENT SUBSTITUTES AND NUTRI...

Core and slice an apple

14 cup mashed avocado, sliced

Blend all of the ingredients together until they're completely dissolved. Serve as soon as possible.

Half the coconut water may be swapped out for greek yoghurt for a richer, protein-rich smoothie. Alternatively, you may add two teaspoons of hemp seeds for protein and make this smoothie plant-based.

Counts as one serving; serving size is one A serving of this meal has 223 calories, 5 grammes of fat, 34 grammes of sugar, and 49 milligrammes of sodium.

Mango and Cilantro Slushie

Cilantro, like coriander, is an excellent source of potassium, calcium, magnesium, and iron, among other minerals. The antibacterial and antifungal properties of this antioxidant-rich plant are a bonus. In any green smoothie that has spinach or kale, add cilantro.

1 litre of coconut water

12 cup of mango that has been frozen Chopped up half a lime and half a cup of cilantro, with the stems removed 1 tbsp. of coconut oil / 2/3 to 1 cup of crushed or cubed ice

There are optional add-ons:

1 cup of kale.

slices of a half-frozen banana

A small amount of spirulina

Amount of avocado: 2 Tablespoons

Blend all of the ingredients together until they're completely dissolved. Serve as soon as possible.

CONVENIENT SUBSTITUTES AND NUTR...

The protein, creaminess, and digestive-supporting probiotics found in Greek yoghurt can all be included in this smoothie, making it an ideal meal replacement.

Counts as one serving; serving size is one 153 calories, 5 grammes of total fat, 27 grammes of sugar, 29 milligrammes of sodium, 30 grammes of carbohydrate, 2 grammes of fibre, and 1 gramme of protein.

Watermelon, ginger, and ginger watermelon cleanse

Watermelon, which is both sweet and hydrating, is an ideal addition for a refreshing and healthy smoothie. Watermelon includes citrulline and arginine, amino acids that can help boost blood flow, as well as fibre, antioxidants, and vitamin C, making it a good source of nutrition.

40 THE COLORFUL SMOOTHIES BOOK

12 ounces of water

Chopped watermelon, 2 cups.

0.5 lbs. peaches frozen

12 lemon juice in 1 cup of kale

12 to 1 cup ice cubes, grated 1 teaspoon fresh ginger

There are optional add-ons:

cup of red or green grapes cayenne

Greek yoghurt, 12 cup

Amount of avocado: 2 Tablespoons

Blend all of the ingredients together until they're completely dissolved. Serve as soon as possible.

Ginger is one of the world's healthiest (and tastiest) spices.

CONVENIENT SUBSTITUTES AND NUTRI...

The fresher the better, but if you're short on time, you may use ground, dried ginger.

Counts as one serving; serving size is one 169 calories; 1 gramme of fat; 26 grammes of sugar; 38 grammes of sodium; 40 grammes of carbohydrates; 4 grammes of fibre; and 5 grammes of protein.

Fennel Apples with a Minty Twist

Fennel is a great addition to green smoothies if you're seeking for something new. Licorice-like fennel is a wonderful source of fibre for heart and colon health because of its diuretic properties. As a source of vitamin C, pectin, and phytochemicals, apples boost flavour and pectin absorption.

1 cup of water.

1 cup of kale.

12 oz. fresh mint, trimmed of stems

Peeled and sliced cucumber

A cored and diced apple

1 cup sliced fennel bulb14 cup chopped avoca-do12 lemon's juice

2/3 to 1 cup of crushed or cubed ice

There are optional add-ons:

12 ice-cold bananas

Ground flaxseed: 2 teaspoons

Minced fresh ginger: 1 tsp.

14 cup chopped fresh parsley

Blend all of the ingredients together until they're completely dissolved. Serve as soon as possible.

Cherry Rooibos Tea

This smoothie's ability to reduce inflammation is out of this world! Quercitin and anthocyanin, two

CONVENIENT SUBSTITUTES AND NUTRI...

powerful pain-relieving and recovery-enhancing phytochemicals found in cherry, may be found in a rooibos tea base. This creamy smoothie is a terrific post-workout drink thanks to the addition of spices.

1 cup rooibos tea, steeped and cooled

Cherries frozen in half a cup

12 cup of frozen papaya

2/3 cup mashed potatoes

2 tbsp. of hemp seed powder

1 tsp. turmeric powder

The equivalent of a half teaspoon of ground ginger

Cinnamon in a sliver

1 tsp. cayenne powder

44 THE COLORFUL SMOOTHIES BOOK

12 cup ice to 12 a pitted Medjool date

There are optional add-ons:

Some 1 to 2 cups of dark greens, or 12 cup of prefrozen greens

12 ice-cold bananas

12-cup bagged blueberries in the freezer

1 tbsp. of coconut oil /

Blend all of the ingredients together until they're completely dissolved. Serve as soon as possible.

Phytochemicals and antioxidants included in teas make them an excellent source of nutrition. Instead of rooibos, try your favourite tea flavour.

Counts as one serving; serving size is one This meal's caloric breakdown is 302, 15g of total fat (15g of which is saturated), 29g of sugar (10g of

CONVENIENT SUBSTITUTES AND NUTRI...

which is fructose, and 10mg of sodium (10mg) of carbohydrate (4g), 8g of fibre, and 8g of protein

Carrots coated with coconut oil

To combat inflammation, "green" doesn't hold all the cards. This smoothie's golden hue comes from the use of golden fruits, vegetables, and spices. In addition to vitamin A, carrots, oranges, and turmeric are all high in vitamin C, potassium, folate, and fibre; they also have anti-inflammatory and healing effects. You'll get the greatest results if you've frozen your orange beforehand.

1 cup of vanilla almond milk, unsweetened Peeled and sliced frozen oranges, one big

12 ice-cold bananas

12 cup grated carrots

1 tbsp. of coconut oil /

46 THE COLORFUL SMOOTHIES BOOK

Chia seeds: 1 tbsp One-half teaspoon turmeric, one-half teaspoon cinnamon, one-half teaspoon cayenne Maple syrup in a half teaspoon 2/3 to 1 cup of crushed or cubed ice

There are optional add-ons:

1 tbsp. coconut shreds

Greek yoghurt, 12 cup

14 cup mashed avocado, sliced

Blend all of the ingredients together until they're completely dissolved. Serve as soon as possible.

It is necessary to freeze your orange in beforehand. A sweet frosty flavour may be achieved by using frozen orange segments that have been quartered and added to citrus smoothies after they have been peeled.

CONVENIENT SUBSTITUTES AND NUTRI...

Counts as one serving; serving size is one 288 calories, 11 grammes of total fat, 30 grammes of sugar, 220 milligrammes of sodium, 49 grammes of carbohydrate, 12 grammes of fibre, and 6 grammes of protein.

Fighter of the Pineapple Cherry Pain

There are several health advantages of eating whole foods, and they can work in conjunction with your body's innate healing mechanisms. Cherry, pineapple, hemp, and ginger are just a few of the potent anti-inflammatory ingredients in this smoothie, so it's perfect for anyone who's been working out hard or who's suffered an injury.

12 ounces of water

12 ounces of tart cherry juice, pure and simple

1 cup of frozen pineapple

48   THE COLORFUL SMOOTHIES BOOK

1-1/2 cups of avocados, diced

Serving Size: 1 scoop of hemp protein powder

Spinach florets in 2 cups

1 tsp. fresh ginger, grated

1 tsp. turmeric powder

1/8 tsp. black pepper, freshly ground

(optional) Stevia (1/2-1 cup) Icing

There are optional add-ons:

12 ice-cold bananas

Chia seeds: 1 tbsp

Cherries frozen in half a cup

Blend all of the ingredients together until they're completely dissolved. Serve as soon as possible.

Hemp protein delivers a more concentrated amount of omega-3 fats, as well as protein and

CONVENIENT SUBSTITUTES AND NUTRI...

fibre, which can help reduce inflammation. 2 tablespoons of hemp seeds can be substituted with hemp protein powder for the same health advantages.

Counts as one serving; serving size is one CALORIE COUNT: 437; TOTAL FAT: 13G; SUGAR CONTENT: 50G; SODIUM CONTENT: 89MG

Inflammation-Reducing Cucumber Arugula

Arugula is a healthy green that lends a spicy taste to smoothies. Arugula is rich in B vitamins and vitamin K, which have been demonstrated to reduce inflammation in the body.

1 cup of water.

Greek yoghurt, 12 cup

1 cup arugula, chopped

1 serving of spinach, chopped finely

50 THE COLORFUL SMOOTHIES BOOK

14 cup cucumbers, chopped

A quarter of a pineapple

12 cup of mango that has been frozen

2 tbsp. almonds / nut

Rolled oats: 1/4 cup

12 tsp. cinnamon powder

Turmeric powder in a half teaspoon measure

The equivalent of a half teaspoon of ground ginger 2/3 to 1 cup of crushed or cubed ice

There are optional add-ons:

14 cup mashed avocado, sliced

2 tblsp. chia seed powder

12 cup of a berry

12 ice-cold bananas

CONVENIENT SUBSTITUTES AND NUTRI...

Blend all of the ingredients together until they're completely dissolved. Serve as soon as possible.

Anti-inflammatory qualities of oats and the addition of texture are the main reasons for their use. If you don't have quinoa, brown rice, millet, or amaranth on hand, you may use any other grain you choose.

Counts as one serving; serving size is one CALORIES: 306; TOTAL FAT: 8; SUGAR: 23; SODIUM: 72; CARBOHYDRATES: 46; FIBER: 8; PROTEIN: 19;

Chia Pineapple Kiwi Spinach

Sweet kiwifruit, a vitamin C powerhouse, has the potential to neutralise free radicals and may help prevent macular degeneration as part of a balanced diet. Vitamin K-rich spinach and omega-3

52 THE COLORFUL SMOOTHIES BOOK

fats round out this smoothie's health-boosting properties.

Almond milk in its unsweetened form

slices of a half-frozen banana

Spinach florets in 2 cups

2 peeled and sliced ripe kiwis

2 tblsp. chia seed powder

1 tbsp. walnuts

12 cup ice to 12 a pitted Medjool date

There are optional add-ons:

Wheatgrass powder in a tablespoon

1 tsp. flaxseed oil

Maca powder: 1 teaspoon

Greek yoghurt, 12 cup

CONVENIENT SUBSTITUTES AND NUTRI...

Blend all of the ingredients together until they're completely dissolved. Serve as soon as possible.

Apply gentle pressure with your thumb and fingertips to choose the kiwifruits that are richest in flavour.

Counts as one serving; serving size is one Three hundred and seventy-one calories, total fat (14g), sugar (37g), salt (233mg), carbohydrate (65g), fibre (16g), protein (10g), and sodium (233mg).

Chapter Four

Diabetes and Loss of Pounds

Blenders make it simple to experiment with a wide variety of ingredients, and the fact that smoothies are so versatile while still being tasty and healthful makes it easy to get carried away. No, that's not entirely correct. Calories in nutritious meals are no different from those in junk food or soda, and they should be treated as such. The good news is that you have complete control over the ingredients you use, and that by following a few simple guidelines, you can create a diabetic smoothie that aids in weight reduc-

DIABETES AND LOSS OF POUNDS

tion. Here are some pointers to remember: When making a smoothie, aim for thick consistency to help you feel full while still consuming fewer calories. Instead of using juices or fruit juice concentrates, opt for low-fat or nonfat milk, water, or coconut water as the liquid. Include protein to help you feel full, as well as fibre and healthy carbohydrates from fruits and vegetables.

Spinach with a Sweet Strawberry Flavor

This smoothie is packed with low-calorie strawberries and slow-digesting protein to help you lose weight. Avocados, which are strong in fibre, and chia seeds, which are high in protein, thicken this smoothie, which gives enough of healthy fats to keep you content for hours.

12 ounces of water

A half cup of nonfat plain Greek yoghurt

THE COLORFUL SMOOTHIES BOOK

Frozen strawberries in a half cup measure

1/4 cup thawed frozen kale (or 2 cups fresh)

Chickpea seeds: 1 tablespoon per serving

2 tblsp. avocado, chopped

Vanilla extract in half a teaspoon Sweetener of choice: Stevia (optional) 2/3 to 1 cup of crushed or cubed ice

There are optional add-ons:

Psyllium husk

1 scoop of your favourite protein powder

Ground cinnamon: 1/4 tsp.

2 tbsp. almonds / nut

Blend all of the ingredients together until they're completely dissolved. Serve as soon as possible.

DIABETES AND LOSS OF POUNDS 57

Adding chia gel to your smoothie will make it more creamy. Chia seeds and water should be mixed together in a small container and left to sit for 15 to 20 minutes before eating. After that, store in the refrigerator for up to a month to use in smoothies.

Counts as one serving; serving size is one There are 191 calories, 6 grammes of total fat, 2 grammes of sugar, 74 milligrammes of sodium, 19 grammes of carbohydrate, 6 grammes of fibre, and 19 grammes of protein in this serving.

Pear with Green Tea Spiced Pear

Two of the greatest natural herbs for weight loss are cayenne pepper and green tea. You may speed up your metabolism and reduce your hunger with the aid of Capsaicin and EGCG, the major active components. Combine the sweet and spicy

58 THE COLORFUL SMOOTHIES BOOK

flavour of chilli powder with pear and banana for a flavorful combination that will please.

a single serving of brewed and cooled green tea

12 cups silken tofu

Chopped slices of a pear with its skin still intact

Slice a half of a frozen banana into rounds.

Ground flaxseed: 2 teaspoons

4 cloves garlic, minced

As much lemon juice as you need 2/3 to 1 cup of crushed or cubed ice

There are optional add-ons:

A small amount of honey 12 cup thawed frozen kale

strawberries in a half cup

DIABETES AND LOSS OF POUNDS 59

Blend all of the ingredients together until they're completely dissolved. Serve as soon as possible.

A supply of protein is essential for satiety and blood sugar stability. If you don't like tofu, just replace Greek yoghurt, cottage cheese, or a scoop of your preferred protein powder.

Counts as one serving; serving size is one Sugars (23g), salts (43mg), carbohydrates (41g), fibre (10) and protein (10) make up the 266 calories in this meal.

a combination of apple and cashew

Fiber, protein, and slow-digesting carbohydrates are all found in plenty in smoothies made with apples and almonds. A kind of fibre found in apples called pectin aids digestion by forming a gel in the stomach and regulating blood sugar levels.

60   THE COLORFUL SMOOTHIES BOOK

Adding creamy cashews to the shake results in a sinfully delicious and satiating beverage.

34 cup of plain soymilk

a single serving of whey protein (whey, hemp, pea, rice, soy)

0.5 lbs. peaches frozen

1 peeled and chopped medium apple

Cashew butter, one-fourth cup

Spice 12-14 cup of ice 14 teaspoon of apple pie

There are optional add-ons:

Frozen spinach in half a cup

1 tsp. flaxseed meal

Extract of vanilla with a teaspoon

CINNAMON SUGAR

DIABETES AND LOSS OF POUNDS 61

Blend all of the ingredients together until they're completely dissolved. Serve as soon as possible.

Cashews can be swapped out for any other nut or nut butter in this recipe. Walnuts, almonds, and pistachios are some of the greatest choices for healthy nourishment. 1 tablespoon of nut butter can be replaced with 2 tablespoons of raw nuts.

Counts as one serving; serving size is one caloric intake, fat grammes, sugar grammes, sodium milligrammes, carbohydrates milligrammes, fibre milligrammes, protein milligrammes

Metabolism Boosting Berries

To make a nutrient-dense and satiating meal, this smoothie includes a generous serving of vitamins, minerals, fibre, protein, and healthy fats. With the sweetness of blueberries and the tanginess of Greek yoghurt, cinnamon has been demonstrated to balance blood sugar levels.

34 cup iced green tea, made as directed.

Greek yoghurt, nonfat, plain, 6oz

Frozen broccoli florets: half a cup

12-cup bagged blueberries in the freezer

1 tsp. flaxseed oil

16 ounces chickpeas

14 cup pistachios, shelled

2 cloves minced garlic, minced 2/3 to 1 cup of crushed or cubed ice

There are optional add-ons:

12 ice-cold bananas

Psyllium husk

1 tsp. ground nutmeg

DIABETES AND LOSS OF POUNDS 63

Blend all of the ingredients together until they're completely dissolved. Serve as soon as possible.

Ground flaxseed can be substituted with the flax oil if you don't have any on hand. You're not quite ready to make a complete commitment? Look for bulk items at your neighbourhood supermarket.

Counts as one serving; serving size is one This meal has 520 calories, 18 grammes of total fat, 29 grammes of sugar, 29 milligrammes of sodium, 68 grammes of carbohydrates, 18 grammes of fibre, and 29 grammes of protein..

White Beans with Mangoes

Beans are a must-have in any diet that aims to help people lose weight or control their diabetes. As a source of long-lasting energy and steady blood sugar levels, beans are an excellent choice. Beans, a smoothie-secret ingredient, contribute

64   THE COLORFUL SMOOTHIES BOOK

smoothness as well as protein, vitamins, and minerals.

Cashew milk, 1 cup

13 cup washed and drained white beans

12 cup of mango that has been frozen

1/4 cup thawed frozen kale (or 2 cups fresh)

2 tbsp. of hemp seed powder

Coconut flour, 1 tbsp.

12 to 1 cup ice, garnished with 2 tablespoons chopped fresh mint leaves

There are optional add-ons:

Greek yoghurt, 12 cup

12 cups silken tofu

1/4 cup gel made from chia seeds

1 tbsp. of coconut oil /

DIABETES AND LOSS OF POUNDS 65

Blend all of the ingredients together until they're completely dissolved. Serve as soon as possible.

In the event that you cannot get cashew milk in your local grocery store, you can use unsweetened almond milk in its place. Soy milk or nonfat dairy milk are good sources of protein.

Counts as one serving; serving size is one caloric intake, fat grammes, sugar grammes, sodium milligrammes (mg), carbohydrates milligrammes (g), fibre milligrammes (g), and protein milligrammes

Raspberry with Peanut Butter

Cherry anthocyanins have been demonstrated to stimulate weight reduction and lessen the chance of developing type 2 diabetes, resembling a peanut butter and jelly taste combo. Enjoy this healthier take on a traditional favourite that's still overflowing with peanut flavour and protein.

THE COLORFUL SMOOTHIES BOOK

The equivalent to 34 cup nonfat milk, soymilk, or protein-fortified almonds milk

12 cups silken tofu

34 cup of frosted cherries

2 tbsp. peanut butter powder

peanut butter, unsalted, about a spoonful

Crush 1 tablespoon psyllium husk with half to one cup of ice cubes

There are optional add-ons:

12 ice-cold bananas

To serve as a garnish, add 1 tablespoon of chopped peanuts.

1/4 cup gel made from chia seeds

CINNAMON SUGAR

DIABETES AND LOSS OF POUNDS

Blend all of the ingredients together until they're completely dissolved. Serve as soon as possible.

PB2 and PBFit are two popular brands of powdered peanut butter. You may get it at your neighbourhood grocer or large box store.

Counts as one serving; serving size is one Caloric intake is calculated as follows: 424; Total Fat 16g; Sugar 22g; Sodium 299mg; Carbohydrate 68g; Fiber 33g; Protein 20 grammes. Calories are divided into five food groups.

Cottage Cheese with Apricots

Cottage cheese and rolled oats provide slow-digesting protein and complex carbohydrates in this smoothie. apricots and raspberries, two of the best fruits for their high-fiber, low-calorie content, give both sweetness and nourishment.

68   THE COLORFUL SMOOTHIES BOOK

This dish is perfect for a substantial breakfast or a satisfying snack in the afternoon.

12 ounces of water

1 1/2 cups of cottage cheese

Two apricots chopped

Frozen raspberries, about a cup

Rolled oats, 2 teaspoons each

Grind 2 teaspoons of flax seed

a Medjool date that has been pitted and chopped
Vanilla extract in half a teaspoon

sugar substitute (optional) half-to-one cup ice

There are optional add-ons:

Frozen spinach in half a cup

1-tbl hemp seed measure

CINNAMON SUGAR

DIABETES AND LOSS OF POUNDS   69

Blend all of the ingredients together until they're completely dissolved. Serve as soon as possible.

Apricots are available from May to August in the United States. In the winter, apricots from South America are imported. Wash, pit, slice, and put them in the freezer while they're in season.

Counts as one serving; serving size is one CALORIES: 489; TOTAL FAT: 9; SUGAR: 51; SODIUM: 465; CARBOHYDRATES: 80; FIBER: 14; PROTEIN: 23;

Avocado with Edamame

For a smooth, sweet smoothie, combine avocado and edamame together. Shelled edamame, often known as green soybeans, is a complete protein, containing all of the body's required amino acids. Protein is a crucial ingredient of any meal, providing fullness, stabilising blood sugar levels, and aiding in weight reduction.

The equivalent to 34 cup nonfat milk, soymilk, or protein-fortified almonds milk

12 cup edamame, shelled

2/3 cup mashed potatoes

12 cup of mango that has been frozen 0.5 tbsp. of coconut meal

(optional) Stevia (1/2-1 cup) Icing

There are optional add-ons:

Frozen spinach in half a cup

1 tsp. flaxseed meal 1/4 cup shredded coconut with 1 teaspoon coconut oil as a garnish

Blend all of the ingredients together until they're completely dissolved. Serve as soon as possible.

DIABETES AND LOSS OF POUNDS 71

Low-carb thickening coconut flour provides fibre and tropical flavour. Almond flour or chia gel can be substituted for the similar consistency.

Counts as one serving; serving size is one caloric intake, fat grammes, sugar grammes, sodium milligrammes, carbohydrates milligrammes, fibre milligrammes, protein milligrammes

The Cocoa Craver

This is great news for chocolate lovers! Fat metabolism and weight reduction may be aided by the polyphenols in dark chocolate. Cocoa is a nonfat component that includes naturally occurring antioxidants without the sugar and fat of chocolate. A healthy approach to satisfy a sweet need without sacrificing taste.

12 ounces of water

Plain Greek yoghurt, 6 ounces

72 THE COLORFUL SMOOTHIES BOOK

Frozen strawberries in a half cup measure

12-cup bag of pre-frozen kale leaves (or 2 cups fresh)

14 cup quinoa boiled with water

1 tbsp chocolate powder, unsweetened

almond butter 1 tbsp.

Chickpea seeds: 1 tablespoon per serving

Vanilla essence, 12 teaspoon, sweetened with stevia (optional) 2/3 to 1 cup of crushed or cubed ice

There are optional add-ons:

Amount of avocado: 2 Tablespoons

Psyllium husk

CINNAMON SUGAR

4 cloves garlic, minced

DIABETES AND LOSS OF POUNDS   73

Blend all of the ingredients together until they're completely dissolved. Serve as soon as possible.

Protein, fibre, and complex carbohydrates are all found in quinoa. Rolled oats, cooked brown rice, or oat bran can be substituted for the same nutritional and textural benefits.

Counts as one serving; serving size is one There are 483 calories in this dish, with 24 grammes of total fat, 16 grammes of sugar, 173 milligrammes of sodium, 54 grammes of carbohydrate, 10 grammes of fibre, and 20 grammes of protein.

Sweet Potato Crust Pie

You're losing out on one of nature's most ideal dishes if you only eat sweet potatoes when they're coated with marshmallows. They're low in calories and high in fibre, making them ideal for those with diabetes. They are packed with

74   THE COLORFUL SMOOTHIES BOOK

nutrients, and their sweet flavour is enhanced by the addition of orange and cinnamon to create a pie-like beverage.

12 cup almond milk, unsweetened

Plain Greek yoghurt, 6 ounces

1 and a half cups of cooked and skinned sweet potato

One peeled tiny orange

12 ice-cold bananas

Rolled oats: 1/4 cup

1 tsp. flaxseed meal

1 tsp. of cinnamon powder (optional) 2/3 to 1 cup of crushed or cubed ice

There are optional add-ons:

1 serving of your favourite protein powder

a teaspoon of hemp seed

Extract of vanilla with a teaspoon

1 tsp. ground nutmeg

A peeled and cored apple

Blend all of the ingredients together until they're completely dissolved. Serve as soon as possible.

You may get equivalent nutrients and flavour using canned pumpkin instead of sweet potatoes. Pick for a pure pumpkin and avoid the stuffing.

Counts as one serving; serving size is one Calories 499; TOTAL FAT: 16g SUGAR: 38g SODIUM 232mg CARBOHYDRATES 77g Fibre 12g Protein 15g

Veggies and Herbs for Weight Loss.

Vitamins and minerals are plentiful in this smoothie since it contains nearly six servings of

76 THE COLORFUL SMOOTHIES BOOK

fruits and vegetables. This smoothie is wonderfully satisfying, thanks to the protein from Greek yoghurt, the fibre from the fruits and vegetables, and the additional flax seed.

1 cup of water.

Plain nonfat Greek yoghurt in a half cup

Cut up 1 cup of romaine lettuce

2 chopped celery stalks

Baby spinach, 2 cups

12 ice-cold bananas

a pear, cored and shaved with the juice of a half-lemon

13 cup fresh cilantro, chopped (can substitute parsley)

12 to 1 cup ice, crushed flaxseed, 1 tablespoon

DIABETES AND LOSS OF POUNDS

There are optional add-ons:

a single serving of a protein powder of your preference

a teaspoon of hemp seed

A peeled and cored apple

Blend all of the ingredients together until they're completely dissolved. Serve as soon as possible.

The cayenne will give you an extra calorie-burning metabolic boost if you use brewed and iced green tea.

Serves 1 | 258 calories, 3 grammes of total fat, 27 grammes of sugar, 124 milligrammes of sodium, 46 grammes of carbohydrate, 10 grammes of fibre, and 16 grammes of protein per serving.

Protein from tropical kiwi and pineapple

78   THE COLORFUL SMOOTHIES BOOK

It will be simpler to make smart eating choices throughout the day if you start the day off with this sweet and creamy smoothie with a tropical flavour. This smoothie is packed with protein, healthy fats, fibre, and vitamins and minerals.

Almond milk that has been fortified with protein

1 cup Greek yoghurt with vanilla flavour, nonfat

1 pound of pineapple

1 medium-sized kiwifruit with its skin still on.

Coconut oil with no added sweetener

6 roasted and blanched almonds

Psyllium husk

12 to 1 cup ice, crushed flaxseed, 1 tablespoon

There are optional add-ons:

1.5-2 cups of leafy leaves in their darkest form

DIABETES AND LOSS OF POUNDS

White beans: 1/4 cup

0.5 tbsp. of coconut meal

Blend all of the ingredients together until they're completely dissolved. Serve as soon as possible.

Nonfat milk or soy milk can be substituted for almond milk that has been protein-fortified. Use water and a scoop of your preferred protein powder instead.

At 537 calories, 11 grammes of fat, 55 grammes of sugar, and 281 milligrammes of sodium per serving, this dish is ideal for one person.

Carbohydrates weigh 105 grammes, fibre weighs 37 grammes, and protein weighs 24 grammes.

Blended Green Tea with Vegetables

Green peas and chia seeds are added to this creamy smoothie for extra protein and fibre and

80 THE COLORFUL SMOOTHIES BOOK

healthy fats, which help keep blood sugar stable and your metabolism revved up. Weight loss-enhancing, calcium-rich Greek yoghurt makes monitoring your waistline taste better than ever..

a single serving of brewed and cooled green tea

Three-quarters cup of low-fat Greek yoghurt

8oz of canned corn

12 cup thawed frozen broccoli

15 ounces canned corn

12 cup of mango that has been frozen

1 frozen banana, 2 tablespoons chia seeds, and stevia (if using)

There are optional add-ons:

The rice bran has been reduced to 1 tablespoon

Rolled oats: 1/4 cup

DIABETES AND LOSS OF POUNDS 81

Leafy greens: 1 to 2 cups

Blend all of the ingredients together until they're completely dissolved. Serve as soon as possible.

Instead of brewing tea, try adding 1 teaspoon of powdered matcha to 1 cup of water for a more potent metabolic stimulant.

Serves 1 | 322 calories, 6 grammes of total fat, 37 grammes of sugar, 168 milligrammes of sodium, 61 grammes of carbohydrate, 15 grammes of fibre, and 18 grammes of protein per serving.

Chapter Five

Dietary Supplementation

Every day, millions of individuals across the world experience digestive problems of some kind. Consuming meals heavy in fat and salt and lacking in fibre can lead to weight gain and health problems. To avoid the need for antacids or other medications, consume an abundance of complete, unprocessed meals. Many fruits and herbs that aid digestion can be found in smoothies, making this a convenient method to get them into your diet on a daily basis. It's easy to receive all the nutrients you need from these beverages

DIETARY SUPPLEMENTATION   83

because they're produced with fresh ingredients then mixed together. In addition to the fiber-rich seeds and fruits of the pectin-rich family like hemp, chia and flaxseed and the probiotic cultured foods of the kefir and yoghurt family like dairy, soy and coconut yoghurt, some of the best meals for digestion include those that are rich in pectin. Among the spices and herbs that aid digestion are fennel (parsley), mint (mint), and ginger (ginger). Try out any of these recipes and see what you come up with.

Chocolate Beets

Unlike yoghurt, kefir is a dairy beverage that is rich in enzymes and has a tangy flavour. Instead than only feeding healthy bacteria, kefir includes helpful microorganisms that colonise the digestive tract. This drink is packed with fibre and

THE COLORFUL SMOOTHIES BOOK

phytochemicals, which will help to relieve your digestive system.

A half-gallon glass of almond milk

12 ounces of kefir

Frozen cranberries in a half cup measure

Bananas that have been frozen

12 cup beets

1 tablespoon cacao or cocoa

2 tbsp. of hemp seed powder

Ice cubes and pitted Medjool dates

There are optional add-ons:

a sprinkling of nutmeg

The powder of acacia is 1 teaspoon

2/3 cup mashed potatoes

DIETARY SUPPLEMENTATION 85

The gel made from chia seeds contains 1 tbsp

Blend all of the ingredients together until they're completely dissolved. Serve as soon as possible.

Buy tiny fresh red beets and cook them unpeeled with a few inches of the tops still attached. Remove the beets' tops and peel off the skins while they are still hot.

Amount of calories: 507; Fat: 14g; Sugar: 65g; SODIUM 210mg; Carbohydrate: 93g; Fibre: 14g; Protein 14g; Per Serving:

Turmeric Lassi That's Easier on the Stomach

This yogurt-based beverage is high in digestive enzymes, friendly bacteria, fibre, and turmeric's anti-inflammatory properties, and is modelled after the traditional Indian beverage. Sprinkle some cardamom on top for an added dose of flavour.

THE COLORFUL SMOOTHIES BOOK

1 cup kefir in its purest form

Papaya frozen in one-cup portions

Freshly grated 2 tablespoons of ginger

Turmeric is one teaspoon

Ground flaxseed: 2 teaspoons

1 tablespoon honey and the juice of half a lemon

There are optional add-ons:

12 ice-cold bananas

2/3 cup mashed potatoes

1 cored and peeled small pear

The gel made from chia seeds contains 1 tbsp

Blend all of the ingredients together until they're completely dissolved. Serve as soon as possible.

Acidophilus yoghurt (and not ordinary yoghurt) can be used in its place if your supermarket does

DIETARY SUPPLEMENTATION   87

not stock plain kefir. Both types include helpful bacteria.

1 | Per Serving: 298 calories; 8 grammes of fat; 25 grammes of sugar; 143 milligrammes of sodium; 41 grammes of carbohydrates; 10 grammes of fibre; and 18 grammes of protein.

Mint Parsley Pineapple

In addition to pineapple, parsley, mint, ginger, and avocado, this electrolyte-rich green smoothie also contains digestive- and immune-supporting ingredients such as pineapple juice and avocado oil. This is an excellent option for breakfast or an afternoon snack because it is light on the stomach. Serve with a wedge of lemon.

12 ounces of water

Coconut water in a half a cup

Pineapple chunks frozen in a cup

88 THE COLORFUL SMOOTHIES BOOK

12 ice-cold bananas

2 tbsp. of hemp seed powder

avo (about two tablespoons)

Fresh parsley in a 14 cup measure

14 cup of freshly harvested mint

0.5 to 1 cup icy water12 to 1 teaspoon of freshly grated ginger

There are optional add-ons:

Probiotic powder: 14 tsp per serving

This recipe calls for 2 cups of dark leafy greens.

honey, about 1 tbsp.

The gel made from chia seeds contains 1 tbsp

Blend all of the ingredients together until they're completely dissolved. Serve as soon as possible.

DIETARY SUPPLEMENTATION 89

Soy yoghurt can be substituted for the water to increase the amount of probiotics. The citric acid in the pineapple may cause kefir and dairy yoghurt to curdle.

455 calories per serving; total fat 13g; SUGAR 64g; SODIUM: 96 mg; carbohydrate 75g; fibre 8g; protein 10g per serving

Smoothie with Avocado and Bananas for Relaxation

This smooth and creamy smoothie is a good bet to ease an upset stomach. Healthy fats and fibre from avocados as well as pectin from bananas promote the formation of good bacteria in the gut. It's so delicious that you'll forget it's good for you, thanks to a foundation of kefir and yoghurt.

12-cup kefir in its purest form

0.5 quarts of unsweetened Greek yoghurt

THE COLORFUL SMOOTHIES BOOK

12 cup chopped avocado

1 sliced frozen banana

Chia seed gel in 2 teaspoons

The vanilla extract, 1 tblsp

honey, 12 to 1 cup, ice, 2 tablespoons

There are optional add-ons:

1-inch cubes of a tiny, peeled and cored apple

a sprinkling of nutmeg

2 tbsp. of hemp seed powder

Blend all of the ingredients together until they're completely dissolved. Serve as soon as possible.

Chia seeds are a "demulcent," a meal that covers and calms your stomach because of the gel they generate when they sit in water. Let it rest for

DIETARY SUPPLEMENTATION 91

15 to 20 minutes with 1 part chia seeds to 1 part water.

Serves 1 | 450 calories, 17 grammes of total fat, 34 grammes of sugar, 116 milligrammes of sodium, 56 grammes of carbohydrate, 11 grammes of fibre, and 22 grammes of protein per serving.

It's a Pear Ginger Digestion Booster

Boosting one's energy levels can be as simple as maintaining a healthy digestive system. GI (gastrointestinal) boosters like ginger and lemon can help improve your digestive health by increasing the amount of fibre in your diet. Pectin-rich pears and creamy avocado provide creaminess to this restorative smoothie.

Plain soy yoghurt in a 1 quart container.

Chopped and cored 1 big pear

1 celery stalk

THE COLORFUL SMOOTHIES BOOK

1 tbsp. freshly grated ginger

2/3 cup mashed potatoes

Spinach florets in 2 cups

1 tsp. flaxseed meal

1 tsp. of lemon juice.

A half to a full cup of ice and 1 tablespoon of honey

There are optional add-ons:

12 ice-cold bananas

The gel made from chia seeds contains 1 tbsp

3 or 4 mint leaves, fresh

Probiotic powder: 14 tsp per serving

Blend all of the ingredients together until they're completely dissolved. Serve as soon as possible.

DIETARY SUPPLEMENTATION 93

The soy yoghurt can be replaced with any sort of cultured yoghurt. L. rhamnosus is the most potent strain of probiotics. bacteria, S. acidophilus Ligusticum thermophilus, Jr. Bifidus, L. bulgar, and bulgar icus. They have casei as an ingredient.

440 calories; 16 grammes of fat; 37 grammes of sugar; 90 milligrammes of sodium; 64 grammes of carbohydrates; 13 grammes of fibre; and 15 grammes of protein per serving.

Extractor of Watermelon

This moisturising and delicious smoothie is built on a foundation of probiotic-rich coconut yoghurt. Watermelon and pineapple are packed with fibre and phytochemicals, and the digestive enzyme bromelain is found in sweet pineapple. This minty smoothie might help keep your digestive system running smoothly.

94 THE COLORFUL SMOOTHIES BOOK

Coconut yoghurt in the form of a cup

1 cup pieces of watermelon

Pineapple frozen in half a cup

Ground flaxseed: 2 teaspoons

mint leaves that have been finely minced

Cinnamon in a sliver

A half to a full cup of ice and 1 tablespoon of honey

There are optional add-ons:

12 ice-cold bananas

Frozen berries: half a cup

1-tbl hemp seed measure

The gel made from chia seeds contains 1 tbsp

Blend all of the ingredients together until they're completely dissolved. Serve as soon as possible.

DIETARY SUPPLEMENTATION 95

Fresh herbs may be frozen and kept on hand at all times. Put the chopped vegetables in ice cube trays, fill with water, and freeze!

Feeds One | Calories: 296; Fat: 13g; Sugars: 33g; Potassium: 203 mg; Carbonates: 50g; Fiber: 16g; Protein: 4g per Serving

Green Apple with Herbs in Pineapple

Smoothie's ingredients all have stomach-calming qualities to soothe your digestive system. In addition to the soothing and coating properties of hemp seeds and honey, pectin-rich apples and enzyme-rich pineapple all contribute soluble fibre and digestion-improving digestive enzymes. Enjoy this stomach soother, which is rounded up with a herbal trifecta.

12 ounces of water

A half-cup of unsweetened soy yoghurt

THE COLORFUL SMOOTHIES BOOK

Pineapple pieces frozen in half a cup

1 cored and diced green apple

1 tbsp. chopped fresh fennel bulb

3 or 4 mint leaves, fresh

Hemp seeds and two tablespoons of juice from a small lemon, plus a tablespoon of fresh ginger

A half to a full cup of ice and 1 tablespoon of honey

There are optional add-ons:

The gel made from chia seeds contains 1 tbsp

a cup of celery, finely chopped

1.5-2 cups of leafy leaves in their darkest form

12 ice-cold bananas

Blend all of the ingredients together until they're completely dissolved. Serve as soon as possible.

DIETARY SUPPLEMENTATION   97

Fennel or anise seeds can be substituted for fresh fennel. Stimulate the growth of beneficial bacteria in your digestive system by steaming fresh artichoke hearts.

440 calories; 11 grammes of fat; 59 grammes of sugar; 32 milligrammes of sodium; 80 grammes of carbohydrates; 11 grammes of fibre; and 13 grammes of protein per serving.

Support for the Blackberry's Stomach

This delicious, creamy smoothie, which is loaded with phytochemicals, vitamins, minerals, and fibre, is a great way to get your required daily fibre consumption started. Bananas and pears provide natural sweetness, while Greek yoghurt adds protein and probiotics for a satisfying start to the day.

A half-gallon glass of almond milk

0.5 quarts of unsweetened Greek yoghurt

98 THE COLORFUL SMOOTHIES BOOK

a half-cup of blackberries frozen

12 ice-cold bananas

a cored and sliced pear

14 cup mashed avocado, sliced

1 tsp. fresh ginger, grated

12 cup ice to 12 a pitted Medjool date

There are optional add-ons:

3 grammes of chia seed gel

2 tbsp. wheat germ flour

Rolled oats, 2 teaspoons each

Hemp seeds: 2 teaspoons

Blend all of the ingredients together until they're completely dissolved. Serve as soon as possible.

Make this a complete dinner by adding one or more of the available add-ins.

DIETARY SUPPLEMENTATION 99

Counts as one serving; serving size is one EX-TRACTS OF CALORIES, TOTAL FAT, SODI-UM, CARBOHYDRATES, FIBER, AND PRO-TEIN:

Stimulant for the Stomach

Probiotics, vitamin C, fibre, vitamins, and minerals are found in plenty in this sweet, earthy-tasting smoothie. Add this to your morning routine and your body will be primed for healthier and simpler digestion throughout the day.

Chapter Six

Lovely recipes

1 cup kefir in its purest form

Frozen strawberries in a half cup measure

12 ice-cold bananas

Cubed 12 cup of cooked and peeled red beets,

Rolled oats: 1/4 cup

Ground flaxseed: 2 teaspoons

Ice cubes to Medjool date12:

There are optional add-ons:

This recipe calls for 2 cups of dark leafy greens.

CINNAMON SUGAR

1 tsp. fresh ginger, grated

Blend all of the ingredients together until they're completely dissolved. Serve as soon as possible.

Compared to red beets, golden or yellow beets are sweeter and have a more mellow flavour. Eat as many golden beets as you can, because they're rich with nutrients!

Counts as one serving; serving size is one Calories: 452; Total Fat: 9g; Sugar: 43g; SODIUM: 196mg; Carbohydrates: 75g; Fiber: 15g; Protein: 22g.

Digestive Ease with Fennel and Melon

Cucumber and melon, both gentle on the digestive tract, work in tandem with digestive support herbs to provide a one-two punch of stomach tranquilly. Detoxify your body with the unusual

THE COLORFUL SMOOTHIES BOOK

flavour and creamy smoothness of this nutritious smoothie.

Plain soy yoghurt in a cup

Chopped melon: 12 cup

12 cups of cucumbers, chopped

12 ice-cold bananas

2 tbsp. of hemp seed powder

Chopped fennel bulb: 1/4 cup

12 to 1 cup ice, 3-4 fresh mint leaves, and

There are optional add-ons:

1 tbsp. fresh ginger grated

1 tsp. flaxseed meal

2 pitted dates Medjool

Chopped fresh parsley: 1 tbsp

LOVELY RECIPES 103

Blend all of the ingredients together until they're completely dissolved. Serve as soon as possible.

Cantaloupe, honeydew, musk melon, or crenshaw are all acceptable melon choices for this dish. In terms of nutritional value, seasonal produce is the best.

Counts as one serving; serving size is one caloric intake, fat grammes, sugar grammes, sodium milligrammes, carbohydrate grammes, fibre grammes, protein grammes

Kefir of Cantaloupe

Probiotics, fibre, and friendly organisms are abundant in this luscious and refreshing smoothie. Vitamins A and C, potassium, fibre, and folic acid are all found in cantaloupe. It also aids with regularity, and its sweet flavour pairs well with

104   THE COLORFUL SMOOTHIES BOOK

creamy banana for a pleasant breakfast or afternoon snack.

1 cup kefir in its purest form

0.5 quarts of unsweetened Greek yoghurt

a cantaloupe, cubed, to make 112 cups

12 ice-cold bananas

Chia seeds: 1 tbsp

Vanilla extract in half a teaspoon 2/3 to 1 cup of crushed or cubed ice

There are optional add-ons:

honey, about 1 tbsp.

1 tsp. flaxseed meal

14 tsp. probiotic strength

Blend all of the ingredients together until they're completely dissolved. Serve as soon as possible.

If your cantaloupes aren't sweet enough, simply add a touch of honey, stevia, or a pitted Medjool date to sweeten things up.

Counts as one serving; serving size is one Amount of calories, total fat, sugar, sodium, carbohydrate, fibre, and protein.

Apple and Banana Spicy

Smoothies like this one, which are easy to make but packed with nutrients and taste great, are a great way to ease digestive problems like indigestion and nausea. More than simply a smoothie component, bananas are a great source of prebiotics, which nourish the good bacteria in your intestines. As part of a healthy diet, eat this frequently.

12 cup almond milk, unsweetened

Acidophilus yoghurt in the form of a half cup

106 THE COLORFUL SMOOTHIES BOOK

The slices of a medium-sized frozen banana

The core and skin of one apple

Rolled oats: 1/4 cup

12 tsp. freshly grated ginger

12 tsp. cinnamon powder

Vanilla extract in half a teaspoon 2/3 to 1 cup of crushed or cubed ice

There are optional add-ons:

1-tblspoon of gel from chia seeds

apple sauce, sweetened or not, to taste

2 pitted dates Medjool

14 tsp. ground cardamom or coriander

Blend all of the ingredients together until they're completely dissolved. Serve as soon as possible.

LOVELY RECIPES 107

Oats can be substituted for brown rice, which is what the BRAT (bananas, brown rice, applesauce, toast) diet calls for.

Counts as one serving; serving size is one CALORIES 384; TOTAL FAT 8; SUGAR 40; SODIUM 151; CARBOHYDRATES 75; FIBER 11; PROTEIN 9G; CALORIES

Chamomile Chamomile Chamomile Chamomile

To soothe the stomach and relax the mind, chamomile tea has been used for centuries in herbal therapy. It is used as the liquid in this stomach-taming smoothie. Relax after a hard exercise or a hectic day with this drink.

Brew and chill one cup of the tea.

Acidophilus yoghurt in the form of a half cup

1 cup of peaches frozen

THE COLORFUL SMOOTHIES BOOK

Rolled oats: 1/4 cup

1 tsp. flaxseed meal

12 tsp. freshly grated ginger

A half to a full cup of ice and 1 tablespoon of honey

There are optional add-ons:

1-tablespoon chamomile dried flowers

Extract of vanilla with a teaspoon

1/4 cup gel made from chia seeds

Blend all of the ingredients together until they're completely dissolved. Serve as soon as possible.

As an alternative, you may prepare the liquid foundation by first steeping two tea bags of chamomile in almond milk in a microwave or on the stovetop for 10 minutes, then chilling for an hour.

Counts as one serving; serving size is one There are 292 calories, 6 grammes of fat, 29 grammes of sugar, 90 milligrammes of sodium, 47 grammes of carbohydrates, 7 grammes of fibre, and 13 grammes of protein in this meal.

Raspberries and Beets with Kale

Beets, which are naturally sweet, are packed with nutrients. The iron-rich kale and the slow-digesting protein in this dish provide you with sustained energy. The inclusion of ginger aids with circulation and provides a natural energy boost, making this a delightful drink.

Soy milk in the amount of half a cup

12 cups silken tofu

a big beet (about 1 cup), cooked, peeled, and diced (approximately 1 tablespoon chia seeds) the juice of 1 orange

THE COLORFUL SMOOTHIES BOOK

Frozen raspberries, about a cup

12 cup thawed frozen kale 1 inch piece of ginger stevia

There are optional add-ons:

Frozen spinach in half a cup

1 tsp. flaxseed meal

Extract of vanilla with a teaspoon

CINNAMON SUGAR

Blend all of the ingredients together until they're completely dissolved. Serve as soon as possible.

Replace the soy milk with orange juice and sweeten with agave syrup and lime juice for a more flavorful and vitamin C-rich beverage (optional).

1 | Per Serving: 385 calories; 8 grammes of fat; 47 grammes of sugar; 181mg of sodium; 69 grammes

of carbohydrate; 13 grammes of dietary fibre; and 16 grammes of protein.

Boost your brain power with berries

Make this brain-boosting smoothie to increase your concentration and memory recall. Choline, a B vitamin found in broccoli, has been linked to improved memory and learning. Antioxidants and omega-3 fatty acids are found in abundance in blueberries and hemp seeds, which help to maintain the health of your brain cells. Add a few brain-boosting extras to make it even better.

12 cup of Apple Juice

Greek yoghurt, 12 cup

a half-cup of blueberries frozen

8oz of canned corn

2 tbsp. of hemp seed powder

0.5 to 1 cup iced tea with 1 spoonful of wheat germ

There are optional add-ons:

1 tbsp. walnuts

1 tbsp. of coconut oil /

0.5 lbs. of finely chopped celery

1/8 tsp tumeric powder

Blend all of the ingredients together until they're completely dissolved. Serve as soon as possible.

Increase the amount of monounsaturated fat in your smoothie by adding 14 cup sliced avocado. Monounsaturated fat is an essential nutrient for brain cell membrane flexibility.

Serves 1 | 333 calories, 8 grammes of total fat, 38 grammes of sugar, 110 milligrammes of sodium,

LOVELY RECIPES 113

54 grammes of carbohydrate, 8 grammes of fibre, and 16 grammes of protein per serving.

Oatmeal with cacao and cacao nibs

To improve our ability to concentrate, we need meals that provide a consistent supply of glucose to the brain. In order to keep your brain in peak condition, oats and soy milk, as well as pumpkin, are excellent sources of energy. Adding cocoa, an ingredient that has been found to increase the flow of blood to the brain, is both sweet and nutrient-dense.

1 quart of soymilk.

a half-cup of pumpkin puree

1 cup of rolled oats

2 tbsp. almonds / nut

Unsweetened cacao or cocoa powder

114 THE COLORFUL SMOOTHIES BOOK

Ice cubes and a handful of pitted Medjool dates

There are optional add-ons:

2 tbsp. cacao nibs, ground

2 tbsp. peanut butter powder

0.5 lbs. peaches frozen

Blend all of the ingredients together until they're completely dissolved. Serve as soon as possible.

If you can't afford dates, you may replace a sweetener of your choice and one tablespoon of chia seeds for a comparable texture.

Serves 1 | 490 calories, 13 grammes of total fat, 47 grammes of sugar, 134 milligrammes of sodium, 85 grammes of carbohydrate, 14 grammes of fibre, and 17 grammes of protein per serving.

Crowdfunding for Strawberry Spinach

LOVELY RECIPES 115

CoQ10 is a naturally occurring antioxidant that aids in energy production, combats free radicals, and may even boost athletic performance. This CoQ10-rich smoothie, produced with some of the greatest dietary sources, is a natural way to up your consumption.

Almond milk in its unsweetened form

Frozen strawberries in a half cup measure

Frozen spinach in half a cup

peanut butter, 1 tbsp.

A teaspoon of sesame oil

Ice cubes and pitted Medjool dates

There are optional add-ons:

A quarter of a cup of chopped pistachios

An orange the size of your thumb

8oz of canned corn

Blend all of the ingredients together until they're completely dissolved. Serve as soon as possible.

With a rich, creamy vanilla taste, rice bran is an excellent addition to smoothies since it is a natural source of CoQ10. In your local supermarket, look for it in the baking or hot cereal section and you'll find it.

Serves 1 | 398 calories, 21 grammes of total fat, 38 grammes of sugar, 267 milligrammes of sodium, 52 grammes of carbohydrate, 9 grammes of fibre, and 10 grammes of protein per serving.

The Papaya Maca Invigorator..

One of the reasons smoothies are so energetic is that they prevent dehydration, which is one of the most common causes of weariness. One of the most critical electrolytes for maintaining

LOVELY RECIPES   117

fluid balance is the potassium found in coconut water. The earthy and nutty flavours of maca, a superfood known for its potential to promote stamina and energy, are a fantastic match for this smoothie.

Coconut water in the amount of 1 cup

14 cup mashed avocado, sliced

12 cup of frozen papaya

Canned Kale: 12 cup

sunflower seeds, about two teaspoons

Maca powder and ice cubes: 1 teaspoon 12 to 1 cup

There are optional add-ons:

Coconut milk in a quarter-cup measure

12 cup silken tofu or Greek yoghurt

THE COLORFUL SMOOTHIES BOOK

1 tbsp. of coconut oil /

Wheatgrass powder in the amount of 1 teaspoon

Blend all of the ingredients together until they're completely dissolved. Serve as soon as possible.

Coconut water and coconut milk are not the same thing. You may get canned coconut milk, which is high in healthy medium-chain triglycerides and includes a large quantity of fat. Increase the creaminess and nutrients by 14 cup.

Prepared for one person | Nutritional Information Per Serving: 178 Calories; 10g Total Fat; 7g Sugar; 16mg Sodium; 19g Carbohydrate; 7g Fiber; 5g Protein

Plants of the Peach Quinoa Pep

Quinoa, soy yoghurt, and hemp seeds make up this smoothie's three complete protein sources. Clean, nutritious fuel for your brain and body

LOVELY RECIPES 119

from antioxidants and omega-3 fats, this pleasant and nourishing drink keeps you going all day long.

12 ounces of water

Plain soy yoghurt, 6 ounces

0.5 lbs. peaches frozen

16 ounces of cooked quinoa 12 cups of frozen spinach

Hemp seeds: 2 teaspoons

Ice cubes and a handful of pitted Medjool dates

There are optional add-ons:

2 tbsp. peanut butter powder

14 cup edamame, shelled

almond butter 1 tbsp.

Blend all of the ingredients together until they're completely dissolved. Serve as soon as possible.

120 THE COLORFUL SMOOTHIES BOOK

You may prepare grains in quantity on the weekends and store the portions you don't use right away in the refrigerator or freezer. Preparing your meals ahead of time might save you a lot of time on a hectic morning.

Calories: 474; Total Fat: 13g, SUGAR: 52g; SODIUM: 28mg; CARBOHYDRATES: 78; FIBER: 8g, PROTEIN: 18g per serving

Infused Seeds Blackberry Broccoli Blackberry

Blackberries, broccoli, and pumpkin seeds are packed with vitamins C and K, which aid mental agility, and zinc, which aids memory and thinking. Cottage cheese, which is strong in protein, helps you feel full, while whole-grain oats keep your brain well-fueled.

34 cup of almond milk that has not been sweetened

LOVELY RECIPES 121

1 1/2 cups of cottage cheese

a half-cup of blackberries frozen

8oz of canned corn

This recipe calls for 1 cup oats, 1 cup pumpkin seeds, and 1 teaspoon stevia (optional).

There are optional add-ons:

Frozen spinach in half a cup

12 ice-cold bananas

Chia seeds: 1 tbsp

Blend all of the ingredients together until they're completely dissolved. Serve as soon as possible.

To up the antioxidants, caffeine, and metabolism-boosting EGCG in your drink, swap out the almond milk for green tea and top with a squeeze of lemon and honey.

122 THE COLORFUL SMOOTHIES BOOK

There are 473 calories per serving, 23 grammes of fat, 9 grammes of sugars, 618 milligrammes sulphate in the salty soup and 42 grammes of carbohydrates, 13 grammes of fibre, and 31 grammes of protein.

Sunrise of Strawberry

Pomegranate juice adds a burst of colour and a distinct flavour to this smoothie. Pomegranate juice's antioxidants may enhance blood flow, particularly to the heart and brain, giving it an ideal liquid basis for natural energy and sustenance.

12 ounces of pomegranate juice

Greek yoghurt, 12 cup

Frozen strawberries in a cup

Grind 2 teaspoons of flax seed

1 cup ice cubes 2 teaspoons chopped avocado

LOVELY RECIPES   123

There are optional add-ons:

2 tblsp. of goji berries.

Canned Kale: 12 cup

1-tbl hemp seed measure

Blend all of the ingredients together until they're completely dissolved. Serve as soon as possible.

The antioxidants and phytochemicals in pomegranate juice are fantastic, but if your budget doesn't allow for it, try cranberry, blueberry, or cherry juices instead.

It's a one-person meal, and it has a calorie count of 299, a total fat content of 10 grammes, a sugar content of 27 grammes, and a sodium content of 43 milligrammes.

Delight in the flavour of Java.

124 THE COLORFUL SMOOTHIES BOOK

Dopamine, a neurotransmitter responsible for carrying nerve signals to the brain, is boosted in the body by the nutrients in this smoothie, which helps your body create more of it. Aside from bananas, soy, and almonds, garbanzo beans add magnesium, a mineral that improves blood flow to the brain, to the list of food sources.

34 cup of soy milk

14 cup of brewed and iced coffee with a strong aroma

1 ice-cold banana

16 ounces chickpeas

walnuts in two tablespoonfuls

12 tsp. cinnamon powder

Vanilla extract in half a teaspoon

LOVELY RECIPES 125

1.5-2 cups ice per 1-serving vanilla protein powder

There are optional add-ons:

12-cup bagged blueberries in the freezer

Greek yoghurt, 12 cup

A small amount of spirulina

Amount of avocado: 2 Tablespoons

Blend all of the ingredients together until they're completely dissolved. Serve as soon as possible.

The quality, pricing, and mouthfeel that a protein powder imparts to a smoothie are all highly variable. Before purchasing a large container, buy a few single-serving packets.

Feeds One | Each Serving: 603 Calories; 16g Total Fat; 28g Sugar; 162mg Potassium; 72g Carbohydrates; 15g Fibber; 48g Protein

THE COLORFUL SMOOTHIES BOOK

Cherry Booster

The answer to preparing energy-boosting smoothies is to utilise high-quality, nutrient-dense ingredients, and to balance protein, fibre, and healthy fats in your smoothies. Tofu, nutrient-rich cherry juice, strawberries, and beets make up the foundation of this smoothie, which provides a delightful and natural pick-me-up.

12 ounces of tart cherry juice, pure and simple

12 cups silken tofu

Cherries frozen in half a cup

Frozen cranberries in a half cup measure

Raw or roasted beets, cut into cubes, 13 cup

12 ice-cold bananas

Hemp seeds: 2 teaspoons

0.5 to 1 cup icy water 1 tablespoon wheat germ 1 teaspoon grated ginger stevia (optional)

There are optional add-ons:

An avocado with a quarter of it.

Core and slice an apple

1.5-2 cups of leafy leaves in their darkest form

Maca powder: 1 teaspoon

Blend all of the ingredients together until they're completely dissolved. Serve as soon as possible.

Pomegranate and cranberry juices are also high in nutrients and might be substituted. You have the option of customising the berries to suit your tastes.

430 calories; 11 grammes of fat; 48 grammes of sugar; 196 milligrammes of sodium; 71 grammes

128 THE COLORFUL SMOOTHIES BOOK

of carbohydrates; 11 grammes of fibre; and 18 grammes of protein per serving.

Beans of the Pinto family, chocolate

If you don't have time to make a cup of coffee, this smoothie is an excellent substitute. If you're in need of a little additional energy, this protein and fiber-packed smoothie is precisely what you need.

12 cup of vanilla almond milk that is unsweetened

Greek yoghurt, 12 cup

12-cup bagged blueberries in the freezer

12 ice-cold bananas

2 tbsp. of avocado chopped

Pinto beans, 12 cup

A pitted date that has been sliced into small pieces

LOVELY RECIPES 129

Cacao powder, unsweetened, 1 tbsp

Chia seeds: 1 tbsp

1 tbsp. of ground coffee

2 to 1 cup of ice cream with 1 teaspoon vanilla extract

There are optional add-ons:

Wheat germ is a tablespoon.

1.5-2 cups of leafy leaves in their darkest form

1 tsp. flaxseed meal

Blend all of the ingredients together until they're completely dissolved. Serve as soon as possible.

Beans of any kind, such as garbanzos, adzukis, black beans, kidney beans, and so on, can be used in this dish. Remove any extra salt by rinsing the beans in a colander.

One serving has 425 calories, 11 grammes of total fat, 25 grammes of sugar, 330 milligrammes of sodium, 66 grammes of carbohydrates, 18 grammes of fibre, and 22 grammes of protein.

The Chard Stabilizer Goji Berry

If your blood sugar levels are out of control, don't worry! Try this slow-burning energy smoothie instead. A flavonoid in Swiss chard has been demonstrated to stabilise blood sugar levels, making it an excellent source of vitamins and minerals. Fruits like goji berries are an excellent source of powerful anti-inflammatory compounds and antioxidants. Cottage cheese and soy milk are good sources of protein that can help you feel energised throughout the day.

Plain soy milk in half a cup

1 1/2 cups of cottage cheese

LOVELY RECIPES 131

2 cups of chopped Swiss chard with the stems removed

Frozen strawberries in a half cup measure

12 cup of pineapple.

cashews, about two teaspoons

1 tsp. flaxseed meal

12 to 1 cup of ice and 1 tbsp of goji berries

There are optional add-ons:

Amount of avocado: 2 Tablespoons

2 pitted dates Medjool

Rolled oats: 1/4 cup

Blend all of the ingredients together until they're completely dissolved. Serve as soon as possible.

Health food stores and huge grocery chains carry dried goji berries. Pomegranate seeds, dried

132 THE COLORFUL SMOOTHIES BOOK

cranberries, cherries, or blueberries are excellent substitutes if you can't locate them.

Serves 1 | Per Serving: 404 calories; 15g fat; 23g sugar; 681mg sulphate, 44g carbohydrate, 8g fibre; 25g protein; 404mg sodium

Protective Immunity

There are several methods to guarantee that your body is getting all the nutrients it needs, and one is to fill your diet with an abundance of fruits, vegetables, clean and lean meats, unrefined grains and healthy fats. A nutritious diet is a necessary for a fully functioning immune system. Avoid processed foods, drink lots of water, get appropriate exercise and rest, take time to relax, and add particular immune-enhancing elements in your diet, such as probiotics, vitamins A, C, B6, E, the minerals selenium and zinc, and a range of phytochemicals. Drinking a smoothie is a convenient, low-cost, and tasty method to obtain your daily dose of essential nutrients to help you stay healthy. In addition, it lowers your chance of developing chronic diseases such as cancer. Here are some delicious dishes for you to try. Choose from a wide range of alternate ingredients and substitutions to match your specific health demands.

Supporting the Immune System with Mango Ginger

These phytochemical- and vitamin C-rich veggies and fruits will give your immune system a much needed boost. Volatile oils in parsley are more than just a pretty garnish; they contain potent antioxidants. This smoothie is packed with nutrients because to ginger's spiciness.

Chapter Seven

Super easy

1 litre of coconut water

1 cup chopped celery

1 cup of fresh parsley

1 sliced and peeled cucumber

1 cup of mango frozen

2 cups of baby kale

1 lemon's worth of grated fresh ginger 2/3 to 1 cup of crushed or cubed ice

There are optional add-ons:

SUPER EASY 135

12 ice-cold bananas 1/2 cup silken tofu with a pinch of cayenne

1 and a half avocados

Blend all of the ingredients together until they're completely dissolved. Serve as soon as possible.

Use your favourite immune-boosting tea in place of the coconut water. Different types of tea, such white, green, black, oolong, and many more, have their own distinct flavours.

To get one serving of this dish, you'll need 296 calories, 1 gramme of fat, 39 grammes of sugar, 340 milligrammes of sodium, and 61 grammes of carbohydrate.

The Immune Boosting Power of Pumpkin and Orange

I'm a huge fan of organic canned pumpkin and purchase it by the case. Oats and smoothies

136 THE COLORFUL SMOOTHIES BOOK

benefit greatly from the addition of this ingredient. Vitamin A and C, betacarotene, and fibre are all found in abundance, so you can't go wrong. Anti-inflammatory spices lend a spicy, warm flavour to this smoothie, making it a great way to start your day.

34 cup of almond milk that has not been sweetened

Orange juice, 14 of a cup

12 cup pureed pumpkin (not pumpkin pie mix)

It's one frozen banana that's been cut up

almond butter 1 tbsp.

1 tsp. flaxseed meal

1/4 tsp. turmeric powder

Cinnamon powder: 1/4 teaspoon

14 teaspoon of ginger powder (or 1 teaspoon fresh)

12 cup ice to 12 a pitted Medjool date

There are optional add-ons:

12 cup of soy milk 12 cups silken tofu

Wheat germ is a tablespoon.

Blend all of the ingredients together until they're completely dissolved. Serve as soon as possible.

The pumpkin can be replaced with a cup of loosely packed sweet potato puree (approximately one big potato). Cook for 25-30 minutes at 400 degrees Fahrenheit, then transfer to a blender when they've cooled.

Counts as one serving; serving size is one CALORIE COUNT: 423; SUGAR CONTENT: 40G; SODIUM CONTENT: 149MG; CARBO-

HYDRATE CONTENT: 70G; PROTEIN CON-TENT: 10G

Restart of the Pomegranate

The phytochemicals, antioxidants, and vitamin C in this smoothie will give your body a much-needed pick-me-up. When you're in need of a little additional nutritional boost, whip yourself a batch of this probiotic-rich smoothie.

12 ounces of pomegranate juice

Greek yoghurt, 12 cup

Frozen strawberries in a third cup 1 cup thawed frozen blackberries 1

14 cup of seedless grapes (red or green)

split one kiwi into four equal slices

papaya, sliced into 1-inch cubes, 1/3 cup

Flax oil, 12 tbsp.

SUPER EASY 139

Wheat germ, 12 cup, and ice, 2 teaspoons each

There are optional add-ons:

2/3 cup mashed potatoes

1 to 2 cups dark greens, such as spinach

Chia seeds in two teaspoons

Blend all of the ingredients together until they're completely dissolved. Serve as soon as possible.

Replace the pomegranate juice with antioxidant-rich rooibos tea for a lower sugar content, or add creaminess with dairy alternatives high in vitamin D, such as almond, cashew, soy, or hemp milk.

Per serving, there are 534 calories, 13 grammes of fat, 61 grammes of sugar, 83 milligrammes of sodium, 81 grammes of carbohydrates, 9 grammes of fibre, and 26 grammes of protein.

THE COLORFUL SMOOTHIES BOOK

Boost Your Immunity Using Peanut Butter!

Gut bacteria, which aid in digestion, number in the hundreds. Recent research indicates that a healthy gut is essential for a strong immune system. Vitamins C, B6, D, and zinc are added to this smoothie to help maintain a healthy physique.

1 cup of kefir milk culture

12 cup of soy milk

2 cans of crushed ice 1 cup of frozen strawberries

12 ice-cold bananas

Peanut butter is 2 tablespoons.

Chia seeds: 1 tbsp

Wheat germ is a tablespoon.

12 cup ice to 12 a pitted Medjool date

There are optional add-ons:

1 tsp. flaxseed meal

2/3 cup mashed potatoes

Cinnamon powder: 1/4 teaspoon

Rolled oats: 1/4 cup

Blend all of the ingredients together until they're completely dissolved. Serve as soon as possible.

Soak 14 cup of oats in kefir overnight in the refrigerated to boost the zinc, protein, and fibre content of your smoothie.

Counts as one serving; serving size is one CALORIES: 673; TOTAL FAT: 31; SUGAR: 55; SODIUM: 288; CARBOHYDRATES: 85; FIBER: 16; PROTEIN: 26;

Power of Coconut and Peach

Viruses and colds don't have a chance against this delectable smoothie. The antiviral ingredient lauric acid found in coconut oil enhances the sweetness of creamy peaches. The cashews, oats, and greens in this smoothie, along with the zinc and vitamins A and C they provide, will help you feel your best.

Coconut water in the amount of 1 cup

12 cups silken tofu

6-8 oz. of dark leafy greens, either fresh or frozen

1 cup of peaches frozen

a quarter-cup of roasted cashews

Rolled oats: 1/4 cup

1 tbsp. of coconut oil /

12 cup ice to 12 a pitted Medjool date

There are optional add-ons:

Probiotic powder: 14 tsp per serving

1 tsp. fresh ginger, grated

Coconut grated to a fine powder

Blend all of the ingredients together until they're completely dissolved. Serve as soon as possible.

In order to add smoothness and more lauric acid, one of the medium-chain triglycerides in coconut, substitute light canned coconut milk (not normal, which has much too much fat).

Counts as one serving; serving size is one Calories: 546; Total Fat G;25 SUGAR: 42G; SODIUM: 244MG; CARBOHYDRATES: 63; FIBER: 9G; PROTEIN: 17G;

zinger with raspberry and zinc

Maintaining enough levels of the mineral zinc in your diet is one method to stay healthy throughout the year. Vitamin C and zinc are found in berries, pumpkin seeds, garbanzo beans and

144 THE COLORFUL SMOOTHIES BOOK

cacao. Because zinc can interfere with the absorption of other nutrients, instead of swallowing tablets, try making this tasty smoothie instead.

12 cup almond milk, unsweetened

Soy yoghurt or a half-cup of Greek yoghurt

A one cupful of thawed and frozen raspberries

Amount of avocado: 2 Tablespoons

2 tbsp. roasted pumpkin seed powder

16 ounces chickpeas

cacoa powder, unsweetened, 1 tsp

12 cup ice and 2 pitted Medjool dates

There are optional add-ons:

Wheat germ is a tablespoon.

Pomegranate seeds, about a cup

1.5-2 cups of leafy leaves in their darkest form

Blend all of the ingredients together until they're completely dissolved. Serve as soon as possible.

Zinc and vitamin B6 are both abundant in most beans, both of which aid the immune system. Green peas are a great option for garbanzos if you'd rather live on the edge.

Counts as one serving; serving size is one A CALORIES: 708; A TOTAL FAT: 18G; SUGARS: 88G; AND SODIUM: 146MG

Carbon dioxide: 124g; cellulose: 20g, and whey protein: 23g.

Kombucha with blueberries

Kombucha is a tea-based probiotic beverage that contains helpful microorganisms that aid with digestion and immune function. With good reason, this Asian-inspired beverage has gained popularity across the United States. Blueberries, kale,

146   THE COLORFUL SMOOTHIES BOOK

and ginger combine to create a flavorful smoothie that is packed with antioxidants and vitamins.

Chapter Eight

The lasts

One cup of kombucha

12-cup bagged blueberries in the freezer

A quarter of a cup of avocado

1/2 cup frozen or 12 cup fresh baby kale

2 tblsp. chia seed powder

1 tsp. of ground ginger.

Ice cubes and pitted Medjool dates

There are optional add-ons:

Frozen blueberries, an additional 12 cup

148 THE COLORFUL SMOOTHIES BOOK

1 tbsp. of coconut oil /

2 cloves minced garlic, minced

a one dose of your preferred protein supplement

Blend all of the ingredients together until they're completely dissolved. Serve as soon as possible.

Most stores sell numerous varieties of bottled kombucha, both pasteurised and unpasteurized. You may also use kefir, brewed green or red tea, or Greek yoghurt in place of the yoghurt.

Counts as one serving; serving size is one There are 441 calories in this dish, 15 grammes of fat, 39 grammes of sugar, 82 milligrammes of sodium, 79 grammes of carbohydrate, 15 grammes of fibre, and 10 grammes of protein.

Elixir with Cranberry and Orange

THE LASTS 149

Eating cranberries on a daily basis may help improve the immune system and protect against some cancers. Soy yoghurt provides a probiotic basis for this tangy and sweet smoothie, making it a powerhouse of nourishment.

Soy yoghurt, 1 cup

Frozen cranberries in a half cup measure

12 a watermelon

1 peeled and seeded mini-orange

2/3 cup mashed potatoes

2 tbsp. of hemp seed powder

12 cup ice to 12 a pitted Medjool date

There are optional add-ons:

1 tsp. fresh ginger, grated

1 tsp. flaxseed meal

150 THE COLORFUL SMOOTHIES BOOK

slices of a half-frozen banana

a one dose of your preferred protein supplement

Blend all of the ingredients together until they're completely dissolved. Serve as soon as possible.

During the months of October and November, North American cranberries are in season. When they're in season, stock up and store them in your freezer unwashed for later use.

Counts as one serving; serving size is one Caloric values are as follows: 511; fat total of 20g; sugar 47g; sodium 28mg; carbohydrates 70g; fibre 11g; protein 18g;

Ginger and Cherry Chips

When it comes to cherries, there's not much to dislike. Cherries are packed with nutrients that may help fight cancer, prevent gout, and lower your chance of developing diabetes. Antioxi-

THE LASTS 151

dants, vitamins A, C and D as well as zinc and healthy fats are found in this creamy smoothie.

Greek yoghurt or soy yoghurt, 12 oz.

Coconut water in a half a cup

Cherries in a cup of ice

12 ice-cold bananas

Almonds, 14 cup

Chia seeds in two teaspoons

ginger, grated, 1 teaspoon

To 1 cup ice, add 1 pitted Medjool date12

There are optional add-ons:

12 cup of pineapple.

2 tbsp. of hemp seed powder

Probiotic powder: 14 tsp per serving

152   THE COLORFUL SMOOTHIES BOOK

1.5-2 cups of leafy leaves in their darkest form

Blend all of the ingredients together until they're completely dissolved. Serve as soon as possible.

You may use dairy milk or a nut or plant-based milk in place of the yoghurt and coconut water. If you opt for a plant-based diet, be sure to add some protein back in for extra stamina.

Counts as one serving; serving size is one CALORIES: 504; TOTAL FAT: 21; SUGAR: 51; SODIUM: 93MG; CARBOHYDRATES: 73; FIBER: 15; PROTEIN: 16G

CPSIA information can be obtained
at www.ICGtesting.com
Printed in the USA
BVHW030006070922
646316BV00011B/620